1 Chair Yoga for Seniors Over 60

Chair Yoga for Seniors Over 60

10-Minute Chair Yoga to Enhance Mobility, Shed Weight, and Embrace Aging with Ease Plus a Life-Changing 28-Day Challenge

By Evelyn Gracefeel

Copyright 2024

All rights reserved.

No Part of this cookbook may be reproduced or transmitted in any form or by any means, electronic or mechanical including photocopying, recording, or by any information storage and retrieval system without permission in writing from the publisher.

Your Feedback is Greatly Appreciated

It's through your feedback, support and ratings that I'm able to create the best books possible and serve many more people.

I would be extremely grateful if you could take just few seconds of your time to kindly leave a positive rating of the book on Amazon. Please share positive feedback and ratings for others to see.

To do so, simply find the book on Amazon website and locate the section to drop a review. Select a good rating and drop a positive couple of sentences.

That's it, Thank you so much for your time and support.

Table of Content

Introduction

Welcome to the beginning of a journey towards greater health, vitality, and well-being. Whether you're a seasoned yogi or completely new to the practice, this book is your invitation to discover the incredible benefits of chair yoga specifically tailored for seniors over 60.

As we age, maintaining mobility, strength, and flexibility becomes increasingly important. Chair yoga offers a gentle yet effective way to nurture your body, mind, and spirit, regardless of your fitness level or physical limitations. With the support of a chair, you'll find that yoga becomes accessible to everyone, empowering you to move with ease and grace.

In the pages ahead, you'll learn how chair yoga can:

- Improve joint health and flexibility

- Enhance balance and stability
- Reduce stress and promote relaxation
- Boost energy levels and vitality
- Support weight management and overall well-being

Are you ready to embark on a journey of self-discovery and transformation? Throughout this book, you'll find a comprehensive 28-day chair yoga challenge designed to help you establish a consistent practice, reap the benefits of regular exercise, and cultivate a deeper sense of connection with your body.

Each day, you'll be guided through gentle chair yoga sequences, breathing exercises, and mindfulness practices, all designed to support your physical, mental, and emotional health. Whether you commit to 10 minutes a day or dive deeper into your practice, this challenge offers a roadmap to greater vitality and joy.

So, are you ready to say "yes" to yourself and embrace the gift of chair yoga? Let's embark on this journey together and discover the transformative power of movement, breath, and mindful awareness. Your chair yoga adventure begins now!

Chapter 1: Understanding Chair Yoga

In this chapter, we will delve into the fundamentals of chair yoga, exploring what it is, the myriad benefits it offers for seniors over 60, and essential safety considerations to ensure a safe and enjoyable practice.

What is Chair Yoga?

Chair yoga is a gentle form of yoga that adapts traditional yoga poses to be performed while seated on a chair or using a chair for support. Developed with the specific needs of seniors, individuals with limited mobility, or those recovering from injury in mind, chair yoga offers a safe and accessible way to experience the benefits of yoga without the need for getting down on the floor.

Benefits of Chair Yoga for Seniors

Chair yoga offers a multitude of benefits for seniors over 60, addressing both physical and mental well-being.

i. **Improved Joint Health and Flexibility**: Chair yoga poses gently stretch and mobilize the joints, helping to alleviate stiffness and improve range of motion.

ii. **Enhanced Balance and Stability**: By incorporating poses that focus on stability and core strength, chair yoga helps seniors maintain balance and reduce the risk of falls.

iii. **Stress Reduction and Relaxation**: Chair yoga encourages mindful breathing and relaxation techniques, promoting a sense of calm and reducing stress levels.

iv. **Increased Energy and Vitality**: Regular chair yoga practice can help boost energy levels, leaving you feeling more vibrant and revitalized.

v. **Support for Weight Management**: Chair yoga promotes gentle movement and mindfulness around eating habits, supporting healthy weight management.

vi. **Community and Connection**: Chair yoga classes provide an opportunity for seniors to connect with others in a supportive and welcoming environment, fostering a sense of community and belonging.

Safety Considerations and Precautions

While chair yoga is generally safe for most seniors, it's essential to approach the practice with mindfulness and attention to individual needs.

a. **Listen to Your Body**: Pay attention to how your body feels during practice and honor your limits. Avoid any movements that cause pain or discomfort.

b. **Use Props and Modifications**: Utilize props such as blocks or cushions to support your practice and make poses more accessible. Don't hesitate to modify poses as needed to suit your abilities and limitations.

c. **Consult Your Healthcare Provider**: If you have any underlying health conditions or concerns, it's always a good idea to consult with your healthcare provider before starting a new exercise program, including chair yoga.

By understanding the principles of chair yoga, recognizing its numerous benefits, and practicing with safety in mind, you'll be well-equipped to embark on a fulfilling and transformative journey towards greater health and vitality.

Chapter 2: Getting Started with Chair Yoga

In this chapter, we'll explore the practical aspects of getting started with chair yoga. From setting up your practice space to selecting the right equipment and ensuring comfort during your practice, you'll find everything you need to begin your chair yoga journey with confidence.

Setting Up Your Practice Space

Creating a dedicated space for your chair yoga practice can help set the tone for a focused and enjoyable experience. Consider the following tips when setting up your practice space:

- **Choose a Quiet and Peaceful Environment**: Select a space in your home that is free from distractions and conducive to relaxation.

- **Clear Clutter and Create Space**: Clear away any clutter or obstacles to create a clean and open area for your practice.

- **Enhances the Ambiance**: Consider adding elements such as soft lighting, calming music, or aromatherapy to enhance the ambiance and create a tranquil atmosphere.

Equipment Needed

One of the beauties of chair yoga is its simplicity and minimal equipment requirements.

✓ **A Sturdy Chair**: Choose a sturdy, stable chair with a flat seat and no arms, if possible. Avoid chairs with wheels or swivel bases, as they may not provide the stability needed for certain poses.

✓ **Comfortable Clothing**: Wear loose, comfortable clothing that allows for ease of movement. Avoid clothing that restricts your range of motion or causes discomfort during practice.

Tips for Getting Comfortable in Your Chair

Ensuring comfort during your chair yoga practice is essential for a positive experience. Follow these tips to help you get comfortable in your chair:

1. **Sit Tall**: Sit up tall with your spine straight and shoulders relaxed. Imagine a string pulling you gently upward from the crown of your head.

2. **Adjust Your Seat**: If needed, add a cushion or folded blanket to your chair to provide additional support and comfort.

3. **Find Your Balance**: Distribute your weight evenly between both hips and feet, grounding down through your sit bones and feet for stability.

4. **Relax Your Muscles**: Relax any tension in your body, particularly in your neck, shoulders, and jaw. Soften your facial muscles and take a few deep breaths to release any remaining tension.

By setting up a comfortable and inviting practice space, selecting the appropriate equipment, and ensuring comfort in your chair, you'll be ready to fully immerse yourself in the transformative practice of chair yoga.

Chapter 3: The Basics of Chair Yoga Poses

In this chapter, we'll explore a variety of foundational chair yoga poses designed to improve flexibility, strength, balance, and stability. Whether you're new to yoga or have been practicing for years, these gentle poses will help you cultivate greater awareness of your body and enhance your overall well-being.

Gentle Stretches and Warm-Ups

Start your chair yoga practice with gentle stretches and warm-ups to awaken your body and prepare it for movement. These movements help increase blood flow to the muscles and joints, reducing the risk of injury and promoting relaxation.

1. **Neck Rolls**: Gently drop your chin to your chest and roll your head from side to side, releasing tension in your

neck and shoulders. Take slow, mindful breaths as you move, allowing your neck muscles to relax with each roll.

2. **Shoulder Rolls**: Roll your shoulders forward and backward in smooth, circular motions, loosening up the muscles in your shoulders and upper back. Focus on keeping your breath steady and your movements fluid as you roll your shoulders.

3. **Arm Stretches**: Extend one arm overhead and gently lean to the opposite side, feeling a stretch along the side of your body. Keep your shoulders relaxed and your spine lengthened as you stretch. Hold each stretch for a few breaths, then switch sides.

Seated Twists and Side Stretches

Seated twists and side stretches are excellent for improving spinal mobility and relieving tension in the back and hips. These poses help increase flexibility in the spine and encourage deeper breathing, promoting relaxation and stress relief.

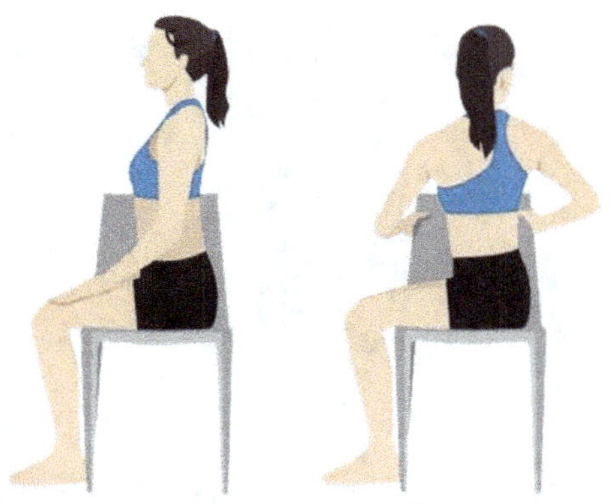

- **Seated Twist**: Sit tall in your chair and place your right hand on the back of the chair. Inhale to lengthen your spine, then exhale to twist gently to the right, placing your left hand on your right knee. Keep your shoulders relaxed and your breath steady as you hold the twist. Take deep breaths into your belly, feeling the twist from your waist up to your shoulders. Hold for a few breaths, then repeat on the other side.

- **Side Stretch**: Sit tall with your feet flat on the floor. Inhale to lengthen your spine, then exhale to reach your right arm overhead and lean gently to the left, feeling a stretch along the right side of your body. Keep both hips grounded on the chair as you stretch, and avoid collapsing into your side. Hold for a few breaths, then switch sides.

Postures for Improving Balance and Stability

Maintaining balance and stability becomes increasingly important as we age. These chair yoga poses will help you strengthen your core and improve your overall balance, reducing the risk of falls and promoting confidence in movement.

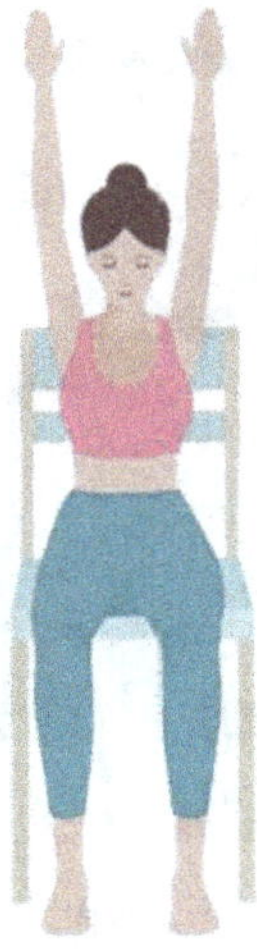

- **Chair Mountain Pose**: Sit tall with your feet hip-width apart and parallel. Press your feet firmly into the ground and reach your arms overhead, palms facing each other. Engage your core muscles and lengthen your spine as you reach upward. Imagine yourself rooted firmly into the ground like a mountain, with your head reaching toward the sky. Hold for a few breaths, feeling strong and stable in your seated mountain pose.

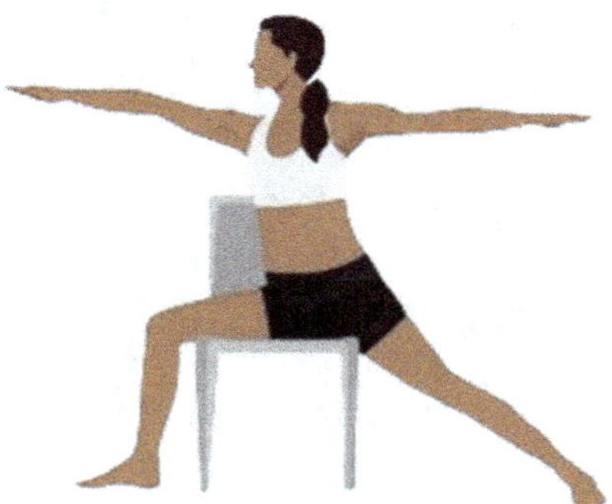

- **Chair Warrior Pose**: Sit sideways on your chair with your right knee bent and your left leg extended behind you. Place your hands on the back of the chair for support. Inhale to lengthen your spine, then exhale to sink deeper into the stretch, feeling a gentle opening in your hips and thighs. Keep your chest lifted and your shoulders relaxed as you hold the pose. Take deep breaths into your belly, feeling the stretch with each exhale. Hold for a few breaths, then switch sides.

By incorporating these basic chair yoga poses into your practice, you'll build strength, flexibility, and balance, allowing you to move with greater ease and confidence in your daily life.

Chapter 4: 10-Minute Chair Yoga Routines

In this chapter, we'll explore three 10-minute chair yoga routines designed to energize you in the morning, provide relaxation during the midday, and wind down your evening with calming stretches. Each routine consists of three exercises, providing a balanced approach to your daily chair yoga practice.

Morning Energizer Routine

Start your day with a burst of energy and vitality with this invigorating morning routine:

1. Seated Sun Salutation

- Sit tall in your chair with your feet hip-width apart and parallel.
- Inhale and reach your arms overhead, palms facing each other.

- Exhale and hinge forward from your hips, bringing your chest towards your thighs.
- Inhale and lengthen your spine forward, lifting your chest and gaze slightly.
- Exhale and fold forward again, bringing your hands towards your feet or the floor.
- Inhale and slowly roll back up to sitting, stacking your vertebrae one by one.
- Repeat the sequence 3 times, moving with your breath.

2. Seated Twist

- Sit tall with your feet flat on the floor and your spine straight.
- Inhale and lengthen your spine, reaching your arms overhead.

- Exhale and twist to the right, placing your left hand on the outside of your right thigh and your right hand on the back of the chair.

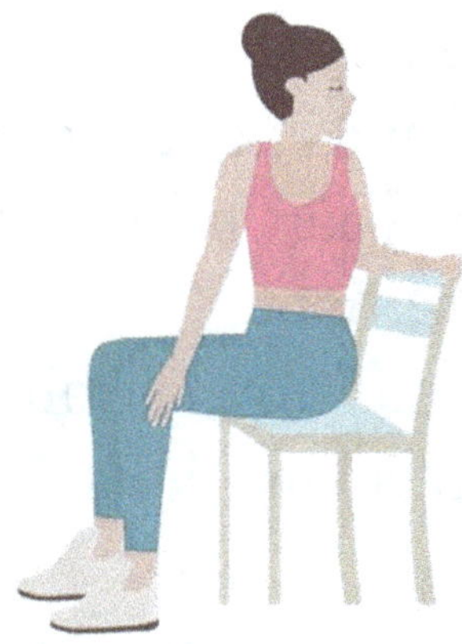

- Inhale and lengthen your spine again, finding space between each vertebra.
- Exhale and deepen the twist, turning your head to look over your right shoulder.
- Hold the twist for 3 deep breaths, feeling the gentle stretch along your spine.

- Repeat on the other side, twisting to the left.

3. Seated Forward Fold
- Sit tall with your feet flat on the floor and your spine straight.
- Inhale and reach your arms overhead, lengthening your spine.
- Exhale and hinge forward from your hips, bringing your chest towards your thighs.

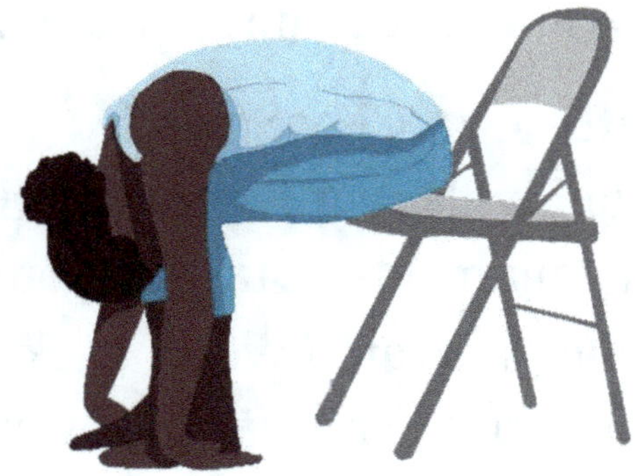

- Allow your hands to come to rest on your shins, ankles, or the floor.

- Keep your spine long and your neck relaxed as you fold forward.
- Hold the forward fold for 3 deep breaths, feeling the stretch along your spine and hamstrings.
- Inhale and slowly roll back up to sitting, stacking your vertebrae one by one.

Midday Relaxation Break

Take a break from your busy day and recharge with this calming midday routine:

1. Seated Cat-Cow Stretch

- Sit tall with your feet flat on the floor and your hands resting on your knees.
- Inhale and arch your back, lifting your chest and gaze towards the ceiling.
- Exhale and round your spine, tucking your chin towards your chest.

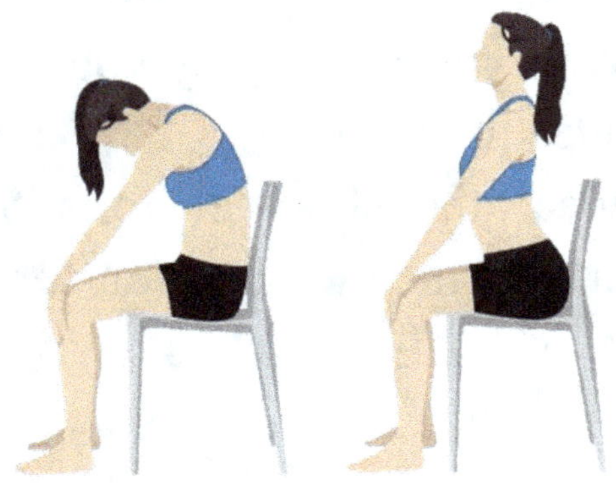

- Continue to move with your breath, flowing smoothly between cat and cow poses.
- Repeat the sequence 5 times, allowing each movement to be slow and mindful.

2. Shoulder Rolls and Neck Stretches

- Sit tall with your shoulders relaxed and your spine straight.
- Inhale and lift your shoulders up towards your ears.

- Exhale and roll your shoulders back and down, squeezing your shoulder blades together.
- Repeat the shoulder rolls 5 times, then reverse the direction for another 5 rolls.

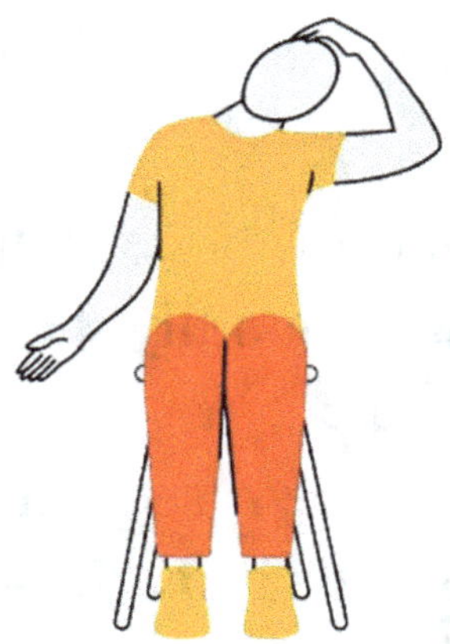

- Inhale and tilt your head to the right, bringing your right ear towards your right shoulder.
- Exhale and release any tension in your neck and shoulder.
- Hold the stretch for 3 deep breaths, then switch sides.

3. Seated Side Stretch

- Sit tall with your feet flat on the floor and your spine straight.
- Inhale and reach your right arm overhead, lengthening your spine.
- Exhale and lean to the left, feeling a stretch along the right side of your body.

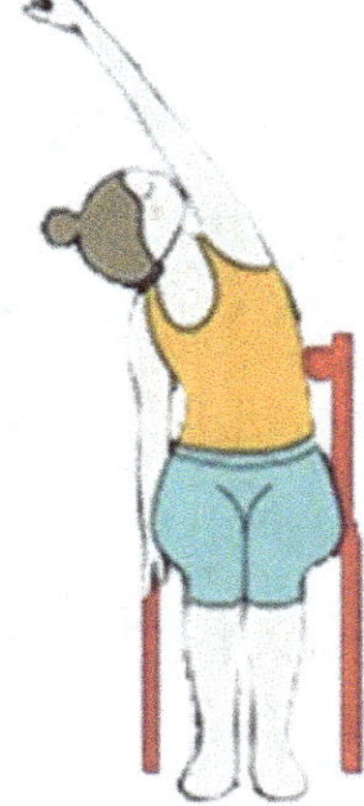

- Keep both hips grounded on the chair as you stretch, and avoid collapsing into your side.

- Hold the stretch for 3 deep breaths, feeling a gentle opening along your right side.
- Inhale and come back to center, then switch sides.

Evening Wind-Down Sequence

End your day on a peaceful note with this soothing evening routine:

1. Seated Spinal Twist

- Sit tall with your feet flat on the floor and your spine straight.
- Inhale and lengthen your spine, reaching your arms overhead.
- Exhale and twist to the right, placing your left hand on the outside of your right thigh and your right hand on the back of the chair.
- Inhale and lengthen your spine again, finding space between each vertebra.

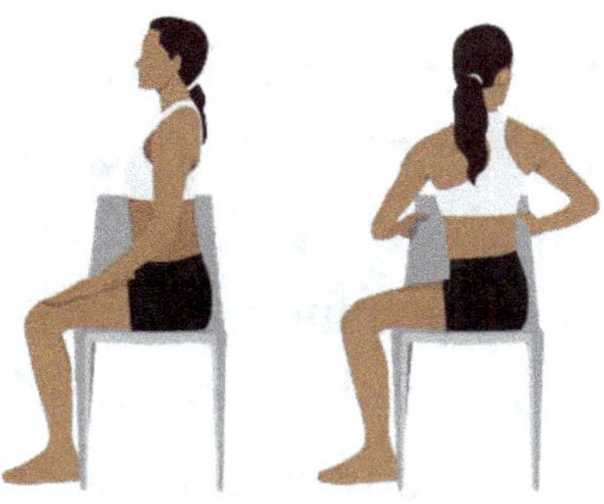

- Exhale and deepen the twist, turning your head to look over your right shoulder.
- Hold the twist for 3 deep breaths, feeling the gentle stretch along your spine.
- Repeat on the other side, twisting to the left.

2. Seated Forward Fold

- Sit tall with your feet flat on the floor and your spine straight.

- Inhale and reach your arms overhead, lengthening your spine.
- Exhale and hinge forward from your hips, bringing your chest towards your thighs.
- Allow your hands to come to rest on your shins, ankles, or the floor.
- Keep your spine long and your neck relaxed as you fold forward.
- Hold the forward fold for 3 deep breaths, feeling the stretch along your spine and hamstrings.
- Inhale and slowly roll back up to sitting, stacking your vertebrae one by one.

3. Seated Relaxation Pose

- Sit comfortably in your chair with your feet flat on the floor and your hands resting on your thighs.

- Close your eyes and take a few deep breaths, allowing your body to relax and unwind.

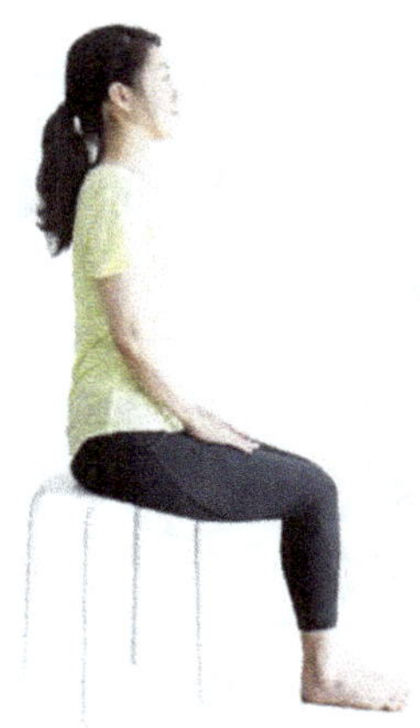

- Scan your body for any areas of tension and consciously release them with each exhale.
- Focus on your breath, allowing it to become slow and steady, like the rise and fall of gentle waves.
- Stay in this seated relaxation pose for as long as you like, allowing yourself

to fully surrender to the present moment.

Chapter 5: Breathing Techniques and Relaxation Practices

In this chapter, we'll explore the power of breath and relaxation techniques to promote calmness, reduce stress, and enhance overall well-being. By incorporating these practices into your chair yoga routine, you'll cultivate a deeper sense of relaxation and inner peace.

Deep Breathing Exercises

Deep breathing exercises are a simple yet effective way to calm the mind, reduce tension in the body, and increase oxygen flow.

1. Abdominal Breathing (Diaphragmatic Breathing)

- Sit tall in your chair with your feet flat on the floor and your hands resting on your abdomen.
- Inhale deeply through your nose, allowing your belly to expand as you fill your lungs with air.
- Exhale slowly through your mouth, gently drawing your navel towards your spine to fully empty your lungs.
- Repeat this deep breathing pattern for several rounds, focusing on the sensation of your breath filling your belly and chest.

2. Equal Breathing (Sama Vritti)

- Sit comfortably in your chair with your spine straight and your hands resting on your knees.
- Inhale deeply through your nose for a count of four.

- Exhale slowly through your nose for a count of four, matching the length of your inhale.
- Repeat this equal breathing pattern for several rounds, maintaining a smooth and steady rhythm.

3. Alternate Nostril Breathing (Nadi Shodhana)

- Sit tall with your spine straight and your left hand resting on your left knee.
- Use your right thumb to close your right nostril, and inhale deeply through your left nostril for a count of four.
- Release your right nostril and use your right ring finger to close your left nostril.
- Exhale slowly through your right nostril for a count of four.

- Inhale through your right nostril for a count of four, then switch sides and exhale through your left nostril.
- Continue this alternate nostril breathing pattern for several rounds, feeling a sense of balance and harmony with each breath.

Guided Relaxation for Stress Relief

Guided relaxation techniques can help release tension from the body and calm the mind, promoting a sense of deep relaxation and inner peace.

Guided Relaxation Script: Progressive Muscle Relaxation

- Find a comfortable seated position in your chair, with your feet flat on the floor and your hands resting in your lap.

- Close your eyes and take a few deep breaths, allowing your body to relax with each exhale.
- Begin to bring your awareness to different parts of your body, starting with your feet.
- Tense the muscles in your feet and toes for a few seconds, then release and relax completely.
- Continue to move up through your body, tensing and releasing each muscle group, including your legs, abdomen, chest, arms, shoulders, neck, and face.
- As you release each muscle group, imagine any tension or stress melting away, leaving you feeling deeply relaxed and at ease.
- Take a few moments to bask in this state of relaxation, allowing yourself to fully surrender to the present moment.

Mindfulness Meditation Techniques

Mindfulness meditation involves bringing your full attention to the present moment, without judgment or attachment to thoughts or sensations.

1. Breath Awareness Meditation

- Sit comfortably in your chair with your spine straight and your hands resting on your knees.
- Close your eyes and bring your attention to your breath, noticing the sensation of air entering and leaving your body.
- Allow your breath to flow naturally, without trying to control or manipulate it in any way.
- Whenever your mind begins to wander, gently bring your focus back

to your breath, using it as an anchor to the present moment.

- Continue this practice for several minutes, allowing yourself to sink deeper into a state of calm awareness.

2. Body Scan Meditation

- Sit comfortably in your chair with your eyes closed and your spine straight.
- Begin to bring your attention to different parts of your body, starting with your toes and slowly moving up through your body to the top of your head.
- Notice any sensations, tension, or discomfort in each area of your body, without trying to change or fix anything.
- As you become aware of each sensation, breathe deeply into that

area, allowing it to soften and relax with each exhale.

- Continue this body scan meditation, moving systematically through your body, until you've scanned every part of yourself.

3. Loving-Kindness Meditation (Metta)

- Sit comfortably in your chair with your eyes closed and your hands resting on your lap.
- Begin by silently repeating phrases of loving-kindness towards yourself, such as "May I be happy, may I be healthy, may I be safe, may I be at ease."
- After a few minutes, extend these wishes of loving-kindness to others, starting with someone you love, then gradually expanding to include

neutral people, difficult people, and finally all beings everywhere.

- Allow the feelings of love and compassion to flow freely, embracing yourself and others with an open heart.
- Sit with these feelings for a few moments, basking in the warmth and interconnectedness of all beings.

Chapter 6: The 28-Day Chair Yoga Challenge

Embark on a transformative journey towards greater health and vitality with the 28-Day Chair Yoga Challenge. In this chapter, we'll dive into the structure of the challenge, daily chair yoga practices, and how to track your progress and celebrate your success along the way.

Overview of the Challenge Structure

The 28-Day Chair Yoga Challenge is designed to help you establish a consistent and rewarding chair yoga practice.

1. **Daily Commitment**: Each day, commit to practicing chair yoga for at least 10 minutes. Whether it's in the morning, afternoon, or evening, carve out time for yourself to nourish your body, mind, and spirit.

2. **Progressive Sequences**: Throughout the challenge, you'll gradually build upon your practice with progressive sequences designed to increase flexibility, strength, and balance.

3. **Mindfulness Integration**: In addition to physical poses, each practice will incorporate mindfulness techniques such as deep breathing, relaxation, and meditation to promote holistic well-being.

4. **Community Support**: Joining the challenge means becoming part of a supportive community of individuals who share your commitment to health and wellness. Connect with others, share your experiences, and cheer each other on throughout the journey.

Daily Chair Yoga Practices

Each day of the challenge will feature a unique chair yoga practice tailored to address different aspects of your well-being.

- **Morning Energizer**: Start your day with gentle stretches and energizing breathwork to awaken your body and mind, setting a positive tone for the day ahead.

- **Midday Recharge**: Take a break from your busy day to reset and recharge with calming poses and relaxation techniques to relieve stress and tension.

- **Evening Wind-Down**: Wind down your evening with soothing stretches and mindful meditation to promote relaxation and prepare your body for restful sleep.

28-Day Chair Yoga Exercise Plan

Week 1: Foundations

Morning Energizer Routine

1. Seated Sun Salutation:

- Sit tall in your chair with your feet flat on the floor and your hands resting on your knees.
- Inhale and raise your arms overhead, palms facing each other.
- Exhale and bring your palms together, lowering them to heart center.
- Inhale as you raise your arms overhead again.
- Exhale and fold forward from your hips, bringing your hands towards the floor or resting them on your thighs.
- Inhale and lengthen your spine, bringing your hands back to your knees.

- Repeat this sequence for 3 rounds, flowing with your breath.

2. Seated Twist:

- Sit tall in your chair with your feet flat on the floor and your hands resting on your knees.
- Inhale and lengthen your spine.
- Exhale and twist your torso to the right, placing your left hand on your right knee and your right hand on the back of the chair.
- Inhale and lengthen your spine.
- Exhale and deepen the twist, looking over your right shoulder.
- Hold the twist for 3 breaths, then repeat on the left side.

3. Seated Forward Fold:

- Sit tall in your chair with your feet flat on the floor and your hands resting on your knees.
- Inhale and lengthen your spine.
- Exhale and hinge forward from your hips, bringing your chest towards your thighs and your hands towards the floor or resting them on your shins.
- Keep your spine long and your neck relaxed.
- Hold the forward fold for 5 breaths, feeling a gentle stretch in your hamstrings and lower back.

Midday Relaxation Break

1. Seated Cat-Cow Stretch:

- Sit tall in your chair with your feet flat on the floor and your hands resting on your knees.

- Inhale and arch your back, lifting your chest and tilting your pelvis forward (cow pose).
- Exhale and round your spine, tucking your chin towards your chest and tilting your pelvis backward (cat pose).
- Flow between cat and cow poses, syncing your movements with your breath, for 5 rounds.

2. Shoulder Rolls and Neck Stretches:
- Sit tall in your chair with your feet flat on the floor and your hands resting on your thighs.
- Inhale and lift your shoulders up towards your ears.
- Exhale and roll your shoulders back and down, squeezing your shoulder blades together.

- Repeat shoulder rolls for 5 repetitions.
- To stretch your neck, gently drop your right ear towards your right shoulder, feeling a stretch along the left side of your neck.
- Hold for a few breaths, then switch sides.
- Repeat neck stretches for 5 repetitions on each side.

3. Seated Side Stretch:

- Sit tall in your chair with your feet flat on the floor and your hands resting on your knees.
- Inhale and reach your right arm overhead, lengthening your spine.
- Exhale and lean to the left, feeling a stretch along the right side of your torso.
- Keep both hips grounded on the chair.

- Hold the side stretch for 5 breaths, then switch sides.

Evening Wind-Down Sequence
1. Seated Spinal Twist:
- Sit tall in your chair with your feet flat on the floor and your hands resting on your knees.
- Inhale and lengthen your spine.
- Exhale and twist your torso to the right, placing your left hand on your right knee and your right hand on the back of the chair.
- Inhale and lengthen your spine.
- Exhale and deepen the twist, looking over your right shoulder.
- Hold the twist for 5 breaths, then repeat on the left side.

2. Seated Forward Fold:

- Sit tall in your chair with your feet flat on the floor and your hands resting on your knees.
- Inhale and lengthen your spine.
- Exhale and hinge forward from your hips, bringing your chest towards your thighs and your hands towards the floor or resting them on your shins.
- Keep your spine long and your neck relaxed.
- Hold the forward fold for 5 breaths, feeling a gentle stretch in your hamstrings and lower back.

3. Seated Relaxation Pose:

- Sit comfortably in your chair with your feet flat on the floor and your hands resting on your thighs.

- Close your eyes and take a few deep breaths, allowing your body to relax with each exhale.
- Scan your body for any areas of tension, consciously releasing and relaxing each muscle group.
- Allow your breath to become slow and steady, sinking deeper into a state of relaxation with each exhale.
- Remain in the seated relaxation pose for 3 minutes, enjoying the peace and tranquility of the moment.

Week 2: Building Strength

Morning Energizer Routine

1. Seated Mountain Pose:

- Sit tall in your chair with your feet flat on the floor and your hands resting on your thighs.
- Inhale and reach your arms overhead, lengthening your spine.

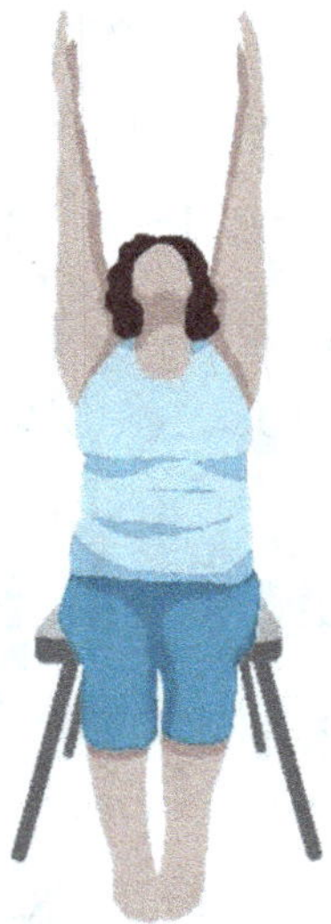

- Exhale and press your palms together, engaging your core muscles.
- Hold the seated mountain pose for 5 breaths, grounding through your feet and lifting through the crown of your head.

2. Chair Warrior Pose:

- Sit tall in your chair with your feet flat on the floor and your hands resting on your thighs.
- Inhale and extend your arms overhead, palms facing each other.
- Exhale and bend your right knee, bringing it to a 90-degree angle.
- Keep your left leg extended and firmly grounded.
- Hold the chair warrior pose for 5 breaths, feeling strength and stability in your lower body.
- Repeat on the left side.

3. Chair Tree Pose:

- Sit tall in your chair with your feet flat on the floor and your hands resting on your thighs.

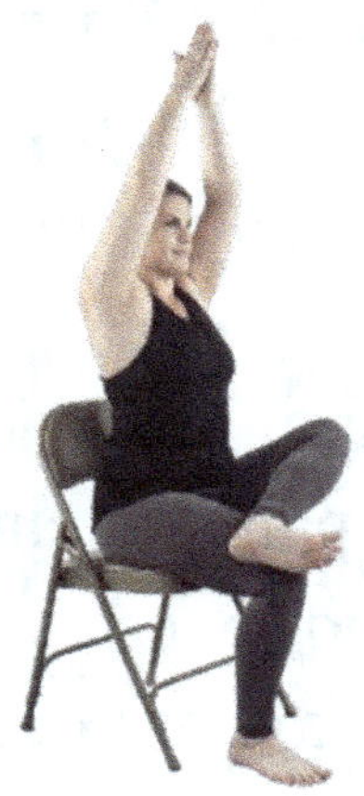

- Inhale and lift your right foot off the floor, placing the sole of your foot on your inner left thigh.
- Press your right foot into your left thigh and your left thigh into your right foot, finding balance and stability.
- Bring your palms together at heart center or extend your arms overhead.
- Hold the chair tree pose for 5 breaths, feeling rooted and grounded through your standing leg.
- Repeat on the left side.

Midday Relaxation Break

1. Seated Forward Fold with Twist:

- Sit tall in your chair with your feet flat on the floor and your hands resting on your thighs.
- Inhale and lengthen your spine.
- Exhale and hinge forward from your hips, bringing your chest towards your thighs and your hands towards the floor or resting them on your shins.
- Inhale and lengthen your spine again.
- Exhale and twist your torso to the right, placing your left hand on your right knee and your right hand on the back of the chair.
- Hold the seated forward fold with twist for 5 breaths, feeling a deep

stretch along the spine and sides of the body.

- Repeat on the left side.

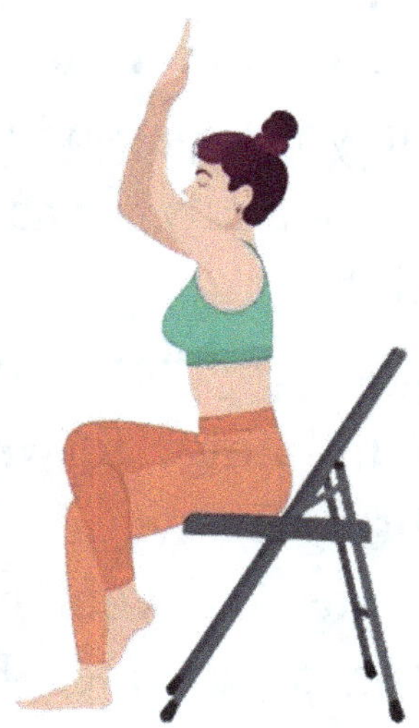

2. Seated Eagle Arms:

- Sit tall in your chair with your feet flat on the floor and your hands resting on your thighs.
- Inhale and reach your arms out to the sides at shoulder height.

- Exhale and cross your right arm over your left, bringing your palms to touch if possible.
- If you can't touch your palms, bring the backs of your hands together or simply bring your elbows towards each other.
- Lift your elbows slightly, feeling a stretch across your upper back and shoulders.
- Hold the seated eagle arms for 5 breaths, then release and repeat with the left arm over the right.

3. Seated Leg Lifts:
- Sit tall in your chair with your feet flat on the floor and your hands resting on your thighs.
- Inhale and engage your core muscles.

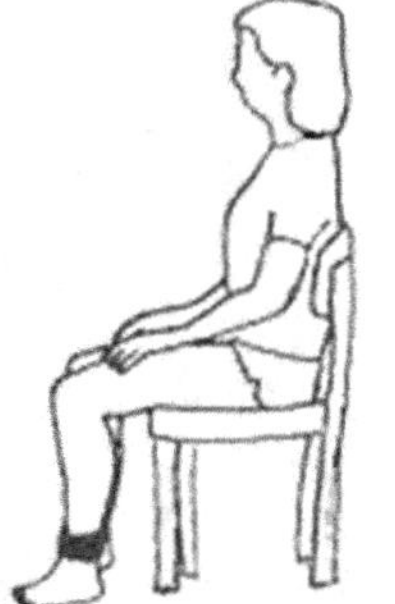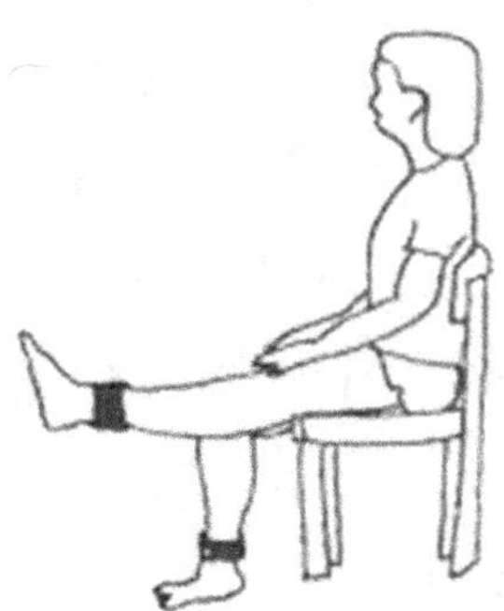

- Exhale and lift your right leg straight out in front of you, keeping your knee straight but not locked.
- Hold the lifted leg for a few breaths, then lower it back down.
- Repeat on the left side.
- Continue alternating leg lifts, aiming for 10 lifts on each side.

Evening Wind-Down Sequence

1. Seated Spinal Twist with Side Bend:

- Sit tall in your chair with your feet flat on the floor and your hands resting on your thighs.
- Inhale and lengthen your spine.

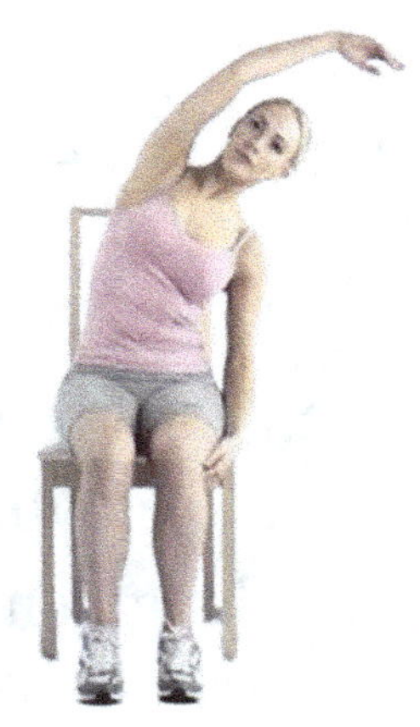

- Exhale and twist your torso to the right, placing your left hand on your right knee and your right hand on the back of the chair.
- Inhale and lengthen your spine again.

- Exhale and lean to the right, feeling a stretch along the left side of your torso.
- Hold the seated spinal twist with side bend for 5 breaths, then repeat on the left side.

2. Seated Wide-Legged Forward Fold:

- Sit tall in your chair with your feet wider than hip-width apart and your hands resting on your thighs.
- Inhale and lengthen your spine.
- Exhale and hinge forward from your hips, bringing your chest towards the floor and your hands towards the floor or resting them on your shins.
- Keep your spine long and your neck relaxed.

- Hold the seated wide-legged forward fold for 5 breaths, feeling a deep stretch in your inner thighs and hamstrings.

3. Seated Relaxation Pose with Belly Breathing:

- Sit comfortably in your chair with your feet flat on the floor and your hands resting on your thighs.
- Close your eyes and take a few deep breaths, allowing your belly to expand with each inhale and contract with each exhale.
- Place one hand on your belly and one hand on your chest.
- Inhale deeply through your nose, feeling your belly rise as you fill your lungs with air.

- Exhale slowly through your nose, feeling your belly fall as you release the breath.
- Continue belly breathing for 3 minutes, focusing on the sensation of your breath moving in and out of your body.

Week 3: Increasing Flexibility

Morning Energizer Routine

1. Seated Cat-Cow Stretch:

- Sit tall in your chair with your feet flat on the floor and your hands resting on your knees.
- Inhale and arch your back, lifting your chest and tilting your pelvis forward (cow pose).
- Exhale and round your spine, tucking your chin towards your chest and tilting your pelvis backward (cat pose).

- Flow between cat and cow poses, syncing your movements with your breath, for 5 rounds.

2. **Seated Side Bend:**
- Sit tall in your chair with your feet flat on the floor and your hands resting on your thighs.
- Inhale and reach your right arm overhead, lengthening your spine.
- Exhale and lean to the left, feeling a stretch along the right side of your torso.
- Keep both hips grounded on the chair.
- Hold the side bend for 5 breaths, then repeat on the other side.

3. Seated Forward Fold with Leg Extension:

- Sit tall in your chair with your feet flat on the floor and your hands resting on your thighs.
- Inhale and lengthen your spine.
- Exhale and hinge forward from your hips, bringing your chest towards your thighs and your hands towards the floor or resting them on your shins.

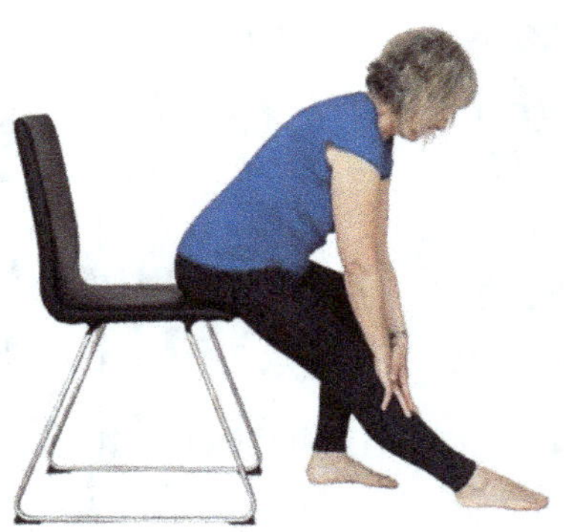

- Keep your spine long and your neck relaxed.
- Extend your right leg out in front of you, flexing your foot.

- Hold the seated forward fold with leg extension for 5 breaths, feeling a stretch in the back of your extended leg.
- Repeat with the left leg.

Midday Relaxation Break

1. Seated Crescent Moon Stretch:

- Sit tall in your chair with your feet flat on the floor and your hands resting on your thighs.
- Inhale and reach your arms overhead, interlocking your fingers and extending your index fingers.

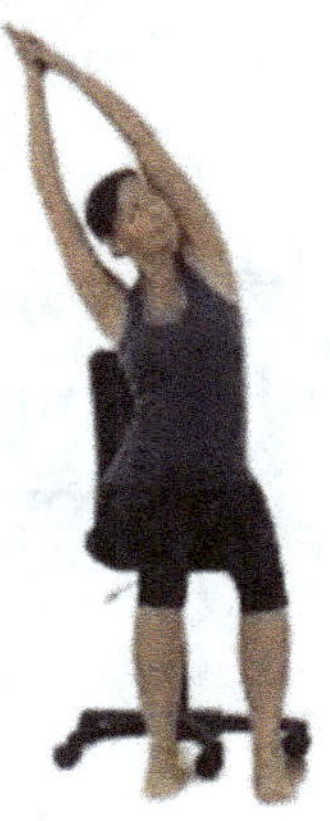

- Exhale and lean to the right, creating a crescent shape with your body.
- Keep both hips grounded on the chair and both shoulders relaxed.
- Hold the seated crescent moon stretch for 5 breaths, feeling a stretch along the left side of your body.
- Repeat on the other side.

2. **Seated Butterfly Stretch**:
- Sit tall in your chair with your feet flat on the floor and your hands resting on your thighs.
- Bring the soles of your feet together, allowing your knees to fall open to the sides.
- Inhale and lengthen your spine.
- Exhale and hinge forward from your hips, bringing your chest towards your feet.

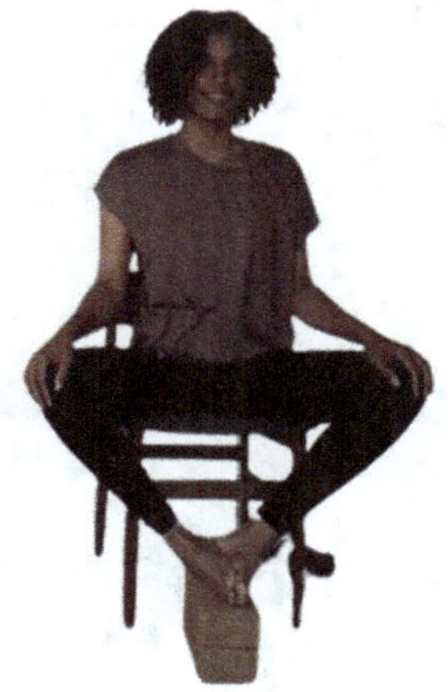

- Keep your spine long and your neck relaxed.
- Hold the seated butterfly stretch for 5 breaths, feeling a gentle stretch in your inner thighs and groin.

3. Seated Pigeon Pose:
- Sit tall in your chair with your feet flat on the floor and your hands resting on your thighs.

- Cross your right ankle over your left thigh, flexing your right foot to protect your knee.
- Inhale and lengthen your spine.

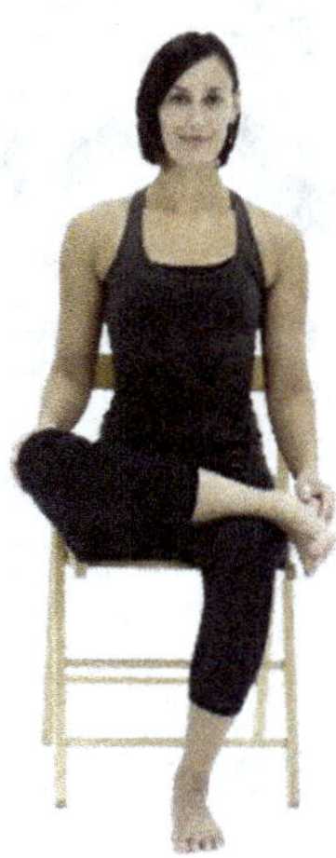

- Exhale and hinge forward from your hips, bringing your chest towards your shins.
- Keep your spine long and your neck relaxed.
- Hold the seated pigeon pose for 5 breaths, feeling a deep stretch in your right hip and glute.

- Repeat with the left ankle crossed over the right thigh.

Evening Wind-Down Sequence
1. Seated Twisting Lunge:
- Sit tall in your chair with your feet flat on the floor and your hands resting on your thighs.
- Inhale and lengthen your spine.
- Exhale and step your right foot back, coming into a lunge position.
- Keep your left knee directly over your left ankle and your right knee hovering off the floor.
- Inhale and lengthen your spine again.
- Exhale and twist your torso to the left, placing your right hand on your left thigh and your left hand on the back of the chair.

- Hold the seated twisting lunge for 5 breaths, feeling a stretch along the front of your right hip and thigh.
- Repeat on the other side.

2. Seated Wide-Legged Forward Fold with Twist:

- Sit tall in your chair with your feet wider than hip-width apart and your hands resting on your thighs.
- Inhale and lengthen your spine.
- Exhale and hinge forward from your hips, bringing your chest towards the floor and your hands towards the floor or resting them on your shins.
- Keep your spine long and your neck relaxed.
- Inhale and lengthen your spine again.
- Exhale and twist your torso to the right, placing your left hand on your

right knee and your right hand on the
back of the chair.

- Hold the seated wide-legged forward
  fold with twist for 5 breaths, feeling a
  deep stretch along the spine and sides
  of the body.
- Repeat on the other side.

**3. Seated Relaxation Pose with Body
Scan Meditation:**

- Sit comfortably in your chair with
  your feet flat on the floor and your
  hands resting on your thighs.
- Close your eyes and take a few deep
  breaths, allowing your body to relax
  with each exhale.
- Begin to scan your body from head to
  toe, noticing any areas of tension or
  discomfort.
- With each exhale, imagine releasing
  and softening those areas, allowing

them to melt into the support of the chair.

- Continue the body scan meditation for 5 minutes, cultivating a sense of deep relaxation and presence.

Week 4: Integration and Flow

Morning Energizer Routine

1. Seated Sun Salutation Flow:

- Sit tall in your chair with your feet flat on the floor and your hands resting on your knees.
- Inhale and reach your arms overhead, palms facing each other.
- Exhale and bring your palms together, lowering them to heart center.
- Inhale as you raise your arms overhead again.

- Exhale and fold forward from your hips, bringing your hands towards the floor or resting them on your thighs.
- Inhale and lengthen your spine, bringing your hands back to your knees.
- Repeat this sequence for 5 rounds, flowing with your breath.

2. Seated Twist with Side Bend:
- Sit tall in your chair with your feet flat on the floor and your hands resting on your thighs.
- Inhale and lengthen your spine.
- Exhale and twist your torso to the right, placing your left hand on your right knee and your right hand on the back of the chair.
- Inhale and lengthen your spine again.

- Exhale and lean to the right, feeling a stretch along the left side of your torso.
- Hold the seated twist with side bend for 5 breaths, then repeat on the left side.

3. Seated Half Moon Pose:
- Sit tall in your chair with your feet flat on the floor and your hands resting on your thighs.
- Inhale and reach your right arm overhead, lengthening your spine.

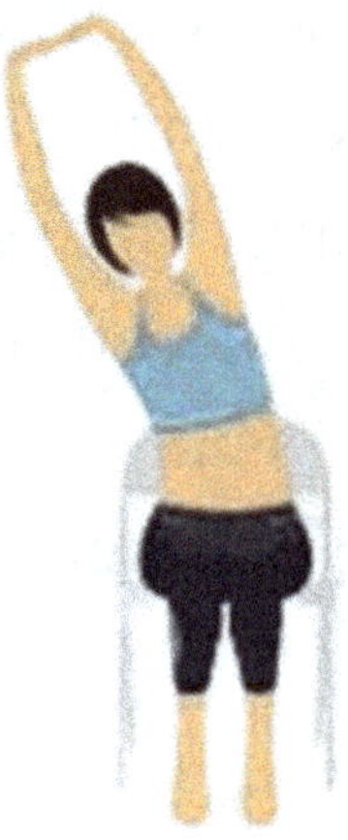

- Exhale and lean to the left, creating a half-moon shape with your body.
- Keep both hips grounded on the chair and both shoulders relaxed.
- Hold the seated half-moon pose for 5 breaths, feeling a stretch along the right side of your body.
- Repeat on the other side.

Midday Relaxation Break

1. **Seated Forward Fold with Shoulder Opener:**
- Sit tall in your chair with your feet flat on the floor and your hands resting on your thighs.
- Inhale and reach your arms overhead, interlocking your fingers and extending your index fingers.
- Exhale and hinge forward from your hips, bringing your chest towards your thighs and your hands towards

the floor or resting them on your shins.

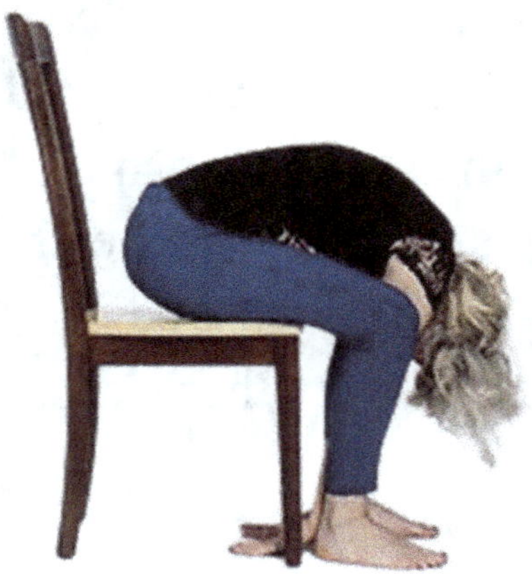

- Keep your spine long and your neck relaxed.
- Hold the seated forward fold with shoulder opener for 5 breaths, feeling a stretch in your upper back and shoulders.

2. Seated Figure Four Stretch:
- Sit tall in your chair with your feet flat on the floor and your hands resting on your thighs.

- Cross your right ankle over your left thigh, flexing your right foot to protect your knee.

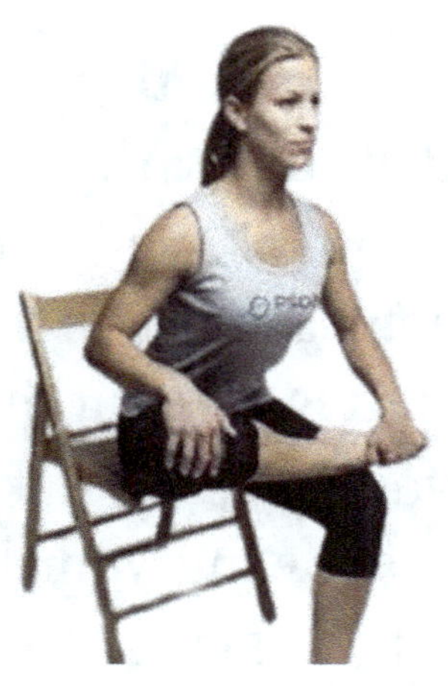

- Inhale and lengthen your spine.
- Exhale and hinge forward from your hips, bringing your chest towards your shins.
- Keep your spine long and your neck relaxed.
- Hold the seated figure four stretch for 5 breaths, feeling a deep stretch in your right hip and glute.

- Repeat with the left ankle crossed over the right thigh.

3. Seated Relaxation Pose with Guided Visualization:

- Sit comfortably in your chair with your feet flat on the floor and your hands resting on your thighs.
- Close your eyes and take a few deep breaths, allowing your body to relax with each exhale.
- Visualize yourself in a peaceful and serene place, such as a beach or a forest.
- Imagine the sights, sounds, and smells of this place, allowing yourself to fully immerse in the experience.
- Stay in this relaxed state for 5 minutes, enjoying the sense of calm and tranquility.

Evening Wind-Down Sequence

1. Seated Spinal Twist with Leg Extension:

- Sit tall in your chair with your feet flat on the floor and your hands resting on your thighs.
- Inhale and lengthen your spine.
- Exhale and twist your torso to the right, placing your left hand on your right knee and your right hand on the back of the chair.
- Inhale and lengthen your spine again.
- Exhale and extend your left leg out in front of you, flexing your foot.
- Hold the seated spinal twist with leg extension for 5 breaths, feeling a stretch along the spine and back of the extended leg.
- Repeat on the other side.

2. Seated Forward Fold with Heart Opener:

- Sit tall in your chair with your feet flat on the floor and your hands resting on your thighs.
- Inhale and reach your arms overhead, interlocking your fingers and extending your index fingers.
- Exhale and hinge forward from your hips, bringing your chest towards your thighs and your hands towards the floor or resting them on your shins.
- Keep your spine long and your neck relaxed.
- Inhale and lengthen your spine again.
- Exhale and lift your chest towards the sky, arching your back slightly and opening your heart.
- Hold the seated forward fold with heart opener for 5 breaths, feeling a stretch in your chest and shoulders.

3. Seated Relaxation Pose with Loving-Kindness Meditation:

- Sit comfortably in your chair with your feet flat on the floor and your hands resting on your thighs.

- Close your eyes and take a few deep breaths, allowing your body to relax with each exhale.

- Bring to mind someone you care about deeply, such as a loved one or a close friend.

- Repeat the following phrases silently or out loud, directing them towards yourself and then towards the person you have in mind: "May I be happy. May I be healthy. May I be safe. May I live with ease."

- Visualize sending feelings of love, compassion, and kindness towards yourself and towards the person you have in mind.

- Stay in this state of loving-kindness for 5 minutes, allowing these feelings to fill your heart and mind.

Tracking Progress and Celebrating Success

Tracking your progress is an essential part of the 28-Day Chair Yoga Challenge, helping you stay accountable and motivated along the way. Here are some tips for tracking your progress and celebrating your success:

1. **Keep a Journal**: Dedicate a journal or notebook to record your daily chair yoga practices, thoughts, feelings, and any insights or reflections that arise.

2. **Set Goals**: Establish specific, measurable goals for yourself at the

beginning of the challenge, whether it's increasing flexibility, reducing stress, or improving balance.

3. **Celebrate Milestones**: Celebrate your achievements and milestones throughout the challenge, whether it's completing your first week of daily practice or noticing improvements in your flexibility and strength.

4. **Share Your Journey**: Share your progress and experiences with the community, whether it's through social media, online forums, or in-person gatherings. Celebrate each other's successes and offer support and encouragement along the way.

Chapter 7: Incorporating Chair Yoga into Daily Life

In this chapter, we'll explore practical tips for integrating chair yoga into your daily routine, ensuring consistency and motivation. Whether you're at home, traveling, or socializing, these strategies will help you maintain a regular chair yoga practice and reap the benefits of improved health and well-being.

Tips for Consistency and Motivation

1. **Set Realistic Goals**: Start small and gradually increase the duration and frequency of your chair yoga practice. Set achievable goals that align with your schedule and lifestyle.

2. **Create a Dedicated Space**: Designate a specific area in your home for chair yoga practice. Keep your chair and any necessary props nearby to make it easy to roll out your mat and start practicing.

3. **Establish a Routine**: Incorporate chair yoga into your daily routine by practicing at the same time each day. Whether it's in the morning to energize your day or in the evening to unwind and relax, consistency is key.

4. **Find Accountability Partners**: Share your chair yoga journey with friends or family members and hold each other accountable. Schedule regular check-ins to discuss your progress and provide support and encouragement.

5. **Celebrate Milestones**: Celebrate your achievements along the way, whether it's completing a week of daily practice or mastering a challenging pose. Acknowledge your progress and reward yourself for your dedication and commitment.

Integrating Chair Yoga into Your Morning and Evening Routines

- **Morning Routine**: Start your day on the right foot by incorporating chair yoga into your morning routine. Set aside time to practice gentle stretches and energizing poses to awaken your body and mind, setting a positive tone for the day ahead.

- **Evening Routine**: Wind down your evenings with calming chair yoga poses and relaxation techniques to release tension and prepare your body for restful sleep. Incorporate gentle stretches, deep breathing exercises, and mindfulness meditation to promote relaxation and inner peace.

Chair Yoga for Travel and Social Gatherings

- **Travel**: Maintain your chair yoga practice while traveling by packing a travel-friendly yoga mat or towel and finding creative ways to practice in your hotel room or at your destination. Focus on simple poses and stretches that don't require much space or equipment.

- **Social Gatherings**: Share the benefits of chair yoga with friends and family by incorporating it into social gatherings. Host a chair yoga session at your next gathering or encourage others to join you in a group practice. Chair yoga can be a fun and inclusive activity for people of all ages and fitness levels.

By integrating chair yoga into your daily life, you'll experience greater consistency, motivation, and overall well-being. Whether you're at home, traveling, or socializing, chair yoga offers a convenient and accessible way to improve your health and vitality.

Conclusion

As you close the final chapter of **"Chair Yoga for Seniors Over 60,"** reflect on the journey you've embarked upon. Throughout this book, you've delved into the transformative practice of chair yoga, discovering its profound benefits for physical health, mental well-being, and overall vitality among seniors.

Within these pages, you've encountered:

a. The foundational principles of chair yoga, including its myriad benefits, safety considerations, and tailored approaches to address the unique needs of aging bodies.

b. Practical techniques and accessible poses to incorporate into your daily routine, from gentle stretches to invigorating flows and soothing relaxation practices.

c. A comprehensive 28-day chair yoga challenge, meticulously crafted to guide you through a transformative journey of self-discovery, growth, and empowerment.

d. Strategies for seamlessly integrating chair yoga into your daily life, from fostering consistency and motivation to seamlessly incorporating it into your morning and evening rituals, as well as navigating chair yoga while on the move or amidst social gatherings.

As you bid adieu to this book, remember that your journey with chair yoga is far from over. It's an ongoing practice—a lifelong companion on your path to holistic well-being.

As you continue along this path:

1. Cultivate patience and self-compassion, embracing each moment of growth and evolution.
2. Listen attentively to the whispers of your body, adapting your practice to meet its ever-changing needs.
3. Embrace each breath, each stretch, and each moment on the mat with gratitude and presence.

Thank you for entrusting me as your guide through "Chair Yoga for Seniors Over 60." May your journey forward be illuminated by the light of inner peace, strength, and joy.

Namaste.

9 798322 705512